I0791178

ISBN: 9781673980967

101

Healthy Eating
Tips & 'Secrets'

Compiled by
NoPaperPress™ staff

CONTENTS

Basic Nutrition Tips & Secrets (5)

Practical Eating Tips & Secrets (7)

Binge Eating Avoidance Tips & Secrets (14)

Eating in Restaurants Tips & Secrets (15)

Eating at Parties Tips & Secrets (16)

Drinking Tips & Secrets (17)

Dessert Tips & Secrets (18)

Weight Control Tips & Secrets (19)

Bonus Tips & Secrets (20)

Related eBooks (23)

NoPaperPress Paperbacks & eBooks (24)

Disclaimer

The following are offered to help you eat in a healthier and more natural way. Use the tips that apply to you – that will help you succeed. Good luck!

Basic Nutrition Tips & Secrets

1) You should consult with a physician before changing your eating habits. The physician should be made aware of and should approve the specific nutritional changes planned.   This is especially true if you have an ailment or a history of medical problems.

2) The diet of most people is not very healthy. Our diets contain too many calories, too much saturated fat, trans fat, cholesterol, added sugar and salt.

3) An understanding of nutrition is not only vital for good health but also helps you control your weight in the long term.

4) Keep a daily food log to record everything you eat. For some people this really works wonders.

5) All foods are a combination of water, carbohydrate, protein, fat and fiber. Knowing this can lead to a better understanding of why a food has a particular caloric value.

6) Water and fiber contain no calories – that is zero Calories per ounce.

7) Protein and carbohydrates are about 4 Calories per gram (110 Calories per ounce) and fat is 9 Calories per gram (260 Calories per ounce).

8) Proteins, carbohydrates and fats are nutrients. Vitamins and minerals are called micronutrients because they are present in foods in much smaller amounts than nutrients. Both are essential to human life.

9) Despite the fact that most adults can get all the vitamins and minerals they need by merely consuming a variety of nutritious foods, many physicians recommend a daily multi-vitamin/mineral supplement as a kind of insurance policy.

10) Many adults over 50 are unable to absorb vitamin B12 in food. People over 50 are able to absorb the synthetic vitamin B12 added to fortified foods and dietary supplements.

11) Phytonutrients, the compounds that give fruits and vegetables their color, are also found in whole grains, dried beans, nuts and seeds. They have many beneficial qualities such as reducing inflammation, acting against viruses, and helping reduce the risk some chronic ailments.

12) Nutritionists define a "junk food" as one that offers little if any essential nutrients – except calories – and when eaten it replaces more important foods.

<u>**Practical Eating Tips & Secrets**</u>

13) In the U.S., we consume more than 100 pounds of sugar per year per person, totaling an unhealthy, nutritionally empty, 500 Calories per day. This large intake of sugar leads to obvious ills, such as obesity and tooth decay.

14) Sugar should be used sparingly by people with low calorie needs and in moderation by most other healthy adults.

15) Contrary to what many believe, the latest scientific evidence indicates diets high in sugar do not cause diabetes. Rather, the evidence indicates that adult-onset diabetes occurs most often in those who are overweight.

16) Thinking about using honey rather than sugar? Honey has about 21 calories per teaspoon while sugar has 15. And the vitamin and mineral content of honey is very low.

17) Free-range animals get more exercise and eat a natural diet, so their meat is usually lower in fat and calories than farm-raised cattle.

18) There is no conclusive evidence that shows that organic food is more nutritious than conventionally grown non-organic food.

19) In the view of many nutritionists, if you can afford it, buy local and organic but you don't have to buy organic across the board because not all organic-labeled products offer added health value.

20) It's worth buying organic for the "dirty dozen": peaches, strawberries, nectarines, apples, spinach, celery, pears, sweet bell peppers, cherries, potatoes, lettuce, and imported grapes. These fragile fruits and vegetables often require more pesticides to fight off bugs

21) Studies have shown vegetarian diets significantly lower the risk of colon cancer, heart disease, high blood pressure and other diseases.

22) Many health care professionals think that eating a healthy vegetarian diet is one of the best things you can do for your short-term and long-term health. But a vegetarian diet must be carefully planned.

23) Drink lots of water – about 8 glasses per day. Try adding a slice of lemon to make it more interesting.

24) Know your daily caloric allowance whether you are trying to maintain your weight or are on a reducing diet. (Again see "Total Fitness - U.S. Edition" by NoPaperPress where you can determine your daily caloric allowance using unique Weight Maintenance tables.)

25) Eat a variety of foods within your caloric allowance, and use the "USDA My Plate" to shape your eating patterns. Try to eat the recommended amount from each food group.

26) When possible, select fresh and natural foods and whole-grain products. Avoid chemical preservatives and additives, artificial and imitation foods, refined and processed foods, and foods that are comprised of "nutritionally-empty calories."

27) Fiber is an important part of a healthy diet. According to the Harvard University School of Public Health, adequate fiber intake reduces your risk of developing various conditions, including heart disease, diabetes, diverticular disease, and constipation.

28) When you eat fiber, it simply passes straight through, untouched by but aiding your digestive system. Zero calories absorbed!

29) Adults should get at least 20 to 35 grams of dietary fiber per day. The best sources are fresh fruits and vegetables, nuts and legumes, and whole-grain foods.

30) For a delicious fiber boost in your diet, try roasted veggies like zucchini and red peppers rather than whole-grain pasta.

31) Most berries (such as blueberries, raspberries) have even more fiber than a comparable weight of most any other fruit.

32) In the United States, for a food to be labeled "whole grain" it must contain more than 51 percent whole grain by weight.

33) Most Americans consume too much sodium (salt). The U.S. Department of Agriculture Dietary Guidelines recommends that healthy adults limit sodium intake to 2,400 mg per day. (One teaspoon of salt contains about 2,300 mg of sodium.)

34) Before you buy, it's important to read and understand the labels on food packages.

35) Protein foods make you feel full longer and a can help you avoid overeating.

36) Nearly every animal food, including dairy products, eggs, meat, poultry and fish are complete proteins because they contain all eight-essential amino acids. Soy is the only plant-based food that has all eight essential-amino acids.

37) Plant-based protein sources lack one or more essential amino acids. Legumes, grains, nuts, and seeds are incomplete proteins.

38) For a complete-protein meal, simply eat any of the incomplete proteins with another but different incomplete protein. Complete proteins result when legumes are eaten with grains, or legumes with nuts or seeds, or grains with nuts or seeds.

39) Harvard Medical School studied egg consumption among 120,000 health professionals with normal cholesterol levels and reported no link between eating eggs and heart disease or stroke.

40) All fish are relatively low-calorie foods and are good sources of protein and fat-soluble vitamins A and D.

41) Oily cold-water fish such as wild salmon, sardines, herring, mackerel and tuna are high in omega-3 essential-fatty acid. Trout also has comparatively high omega-3 content.

42) A downside to eating fish is that some fish are contaminated with mercury, PCBs, dioxins and other environmental pollutants.

43) Large predatory fish such as shark, swordfish, king mackerel and tilefish have the highest concentration of mercury and other environmental contaminates. U.S. Food and Drug Administration advises adults to eat no more than six ounces of high-mercury fish per week.

44) Skinless white-meat chicken and turkey are relatively low calorie, low fat, low cholesterol foods that are powerful sources of high-quality protein, vitamin B_6, riboflavin, niacin, phosphorus and potassium.

45) All soy foods contain a significant amount of plant-based complete protein and omega-3 fatty acid as well as vitamin E, potassium, iron and folate.

46) Carbohydrates provide your body with its basic fuel, the energy your cells need to survive, as well as essential vitamins and minerals, fiber, and other beneficial compounds that promote good health.

47) Fruit and milk are loaded with natural sugar (a carb). But the natural sugar comes with vitamins, minerals (as well as fiber when you eat fruit); whereas the simple sugars in candy, for instance, are nothing but nutritionally-empty calories.

48) Simple sugars require little digestion. When you eat a sweet food, such as a candy bar, your blood sugar level rises rapidly. In response, your pancreas secretes a large amount of insulin. The large insulin response tends to cause your blood sugar to fall to levels that are too low, and in about three hours you feel lethargic and hungry.

49) A relatively new system, called the glycemic index (GI), measures the effect a carbohydrate has on your blood sugar – quantifying how rapidly and to what level your blood sugar rises after you eat a food containing carbohydrates.

50) A candy bar, which is digested rapidly has a high GI and causes an almost immediate jump in your blood sugar; whereas, lentil soup is digested more slowly and has a low GI.

51) The blood lipids cholesterol and triglyceride are found in the plaque on the walls of clogged arteries.

52) Desirable readings for **healthy** individuals are: Total cholesterol level should be less than 200 mg/dl; High-density cholesterol (HDL) should be greater than 40 mg/dl; Low-density cholesterol (LDL) should be less than 130 mg/dl; Triglyceride reading should be less than 150 mg/dl.

53) The latest research seems to show that the total amount of fat in the diet may not be strongly linked with disease. What appears to matter is the type of fat in your diet.

54) Limit your intake of saturated fats. Eat meat less often and fish and poultry more often, and use fat-free or low-fat milk and milk products.

55) Do not eat foods containing partially-hydrogenated vegetable oil because they are high in trans fats. This includes commercially prepared baked goods, snack foods, and processed foods, including most fast foods.

56) Monounsaturated fats "good fats" are derived from plant sources, such as vegetable oils, nuts, and seeds. This type of fat is found in high concentrations in canola, olive and peanut oils.

57) Polyunsaturated fats are also "good fats" and are derived from plant sources, such as vegetable oils, nuts, and seeds, and are in high concentrations in sunflower, soybean and corn oils.

58) Essential-Fatty Acids are a class of polyunsaturated fatty acids that our body cannot create. These fats must be obtained from the food you eat and fall into two groups: omega-3 and omega-6.

59) Omega-3 fatty acids, thought to be heart-protective, are relatively hard to find. Foods high in omega-3 fatty acids are walnuts, tofu, flax seeds and oily fish (salmon, mackerel, sardines, trout and albacore tuna).

60) Omega-6 fatty acids, on the other hand, are more common, easier to find, and are in most oils including sunflower, soybean and corn oils.

61) According to a study published in the Journal of Food Chemistry, broccoli, spinach, kale, Brussels sprouts and other dark green vegetables have the highest cancer-fighting potential found in produce. And all are super-low calorie foods.

62) Steaming in a microwave is an excellent way to cook veggies so they retain nutrients. Another advantage is that steaming adds no fat (calories) or sodium.

63) Hot or cold cereal topped with fruit, and fat-free milk makes a nutritious, relatively low-calorie meal anytime.

64) For a quick low-cal lunch, try a peanut butter sandwich on whole wheat bread with a glass of 1-percent milk and an apple.

65) Keep several bags of your favorite frozen vegetables on hand. Mix any combination of the vegetables, microwave, and top with your favorite light salad dressing. This makes a great low-calorie meal.

66) For another quick low-cal meal, try a Lean Cuisine or Healthy Choice frozen entree with a salad and a glass of 1-percent milk.

67) Keep lean sandwich fixings on hand (whole-wheat bread, sliced turkey, reduced-fat cheese, lettuce, tomatoes and mustard).

68) Try to use mustard on a sandwich instead of mayo.

69) For a healthy and relatively low-calorie meal, buy a veggie sandwich on whole-wheat bread at Subway.

70) If you hate veggies, eat plenty of fruit instead. Fruit is just as healthy and low-calorie as vegetables.

71) Foods loaded with flavor stimulate your taste buds and are more satisfying. So add herbs and spices to your food for a flavor boost and you might not eat as much.

72) Learn to change your eating habits to meet changing activity levels – that is don't eat as much when you're activity level declines.

73) "Eat Slowly." This is especially vital when you're trying to lose weight. If you're someone who eats fast, you're not giving yourself a chance to feel full. While everyone else is still eating, you either sit and pick, or you have seconds, taking in extra calories you could avoid if you would just slow down.

Binge Eating Avoidance Tips & Secrets

74) Most nutritionists recommend that you eat a substantial breakfast because then you'll likely eat less the remainder of the day.

75) Eating late at night doesn't by itself cause weight gain. This is because it's the total number of calories that count – not when you eat them.

76) But don't "snack" yourself fat. You can easily munch 600 calories of chips and dips while watching late-night TV.

77) A majority of people who struggle with night binge eating are those who skip meals during the day. Make sure you eat breakfast, lunch, and dinner.

78) To avoid night-time binge eating, change your evening routine.   Rather than watching TV get into a hobby that will occupy your mind and hands.

79) Post a notice on your kitchen and refrigerator doors: "Closed After Dinner."

80) Try brushing your teeth immediately after dinner to discourage you from continued night-time eating.

<u>**Eating in Restaurants Tips & Secrets**</u>

81) Eating in a restaurant can be a challenge because most restaurant portions are huge, and can easily total more than 1,500 Calories.   So, when you're in a restaurant decide how much to eat – and take the remainder home. A good rule of thumb is to eat half and bring the rest home.

82) When you're eating out, consider ordering children's portions or a small sandwich as a way to trim calories and get the size of your meals under control.

83) In a restaurant, consider ordering two appetizers (one should be low-calorie) instead of an entrée, and always request sauces and dressings on the side.

84) For better calorie control, eat at home rather than in a restaurant.

85) For better control over what you eat bring your lunch to work.

<u>**Eating at Parties Tips & Secrets**</u>
86) Before you go to a party, have a very small meal or snack. This will take the edge off your appetite and make it easier to resist high-calorie goodies.

87) At a party, don't stand near temptation – the food and bar! Make an effort, and you'll find you might eat and drink less.

88) If you host a dinner party, when company leaves, have them take some of the leftover food (particularly the dessert) with them – or take the leftovers to work the next day.

Drinking Tips & Secrets

89) Wine and beer contain a small amount of nutrients and micronutrients, but other alcoholic beverages, such as

whiskey, vodka and gin consist of nothing but "nutritionally-empty calories."

90) Beer has about 13 Calories per ounce, wine has 25 Calories per ounce and whiskey has a whopping 71 Calories per ounce!

91) Drink alcoholic beverages in moderation and try to restrict any alcoholic drinking to weekends.

92) Stop drinking your calories. Alcoholic drinks, fancy coffees, regular soda, and even fruit juice are high in calories – but they don't make you feel full.

93) Dilute fruit juices, such as apple juice, orange juice, etc. with water. This does cut the flavor slightly but really reduces the calorie content.

94) Caffeine should be used in moderation. Caffeine is found in coffee, tea, some soft drinks and foods that contain cocoa. It is also in some drugs such as cold remedies and in medicine sold over the counter to relieve headaches.

<u>**Dessert Tips & Secrets**</u>
95) Don't have sweets in your home. This makes them easier to resist. Out of sight, out of mind!

96) Instead of sweets, for a delicious, healthy, low-calorie dessert have a low-cal smoothie, or sliced fruit over low-fat or fat-free yogurt.

97) Not eating your favorite foods sometimes triggers "rebound" overeating. Even on a diet you can still enjoy your favorite foods, but do so in moderation.

98) If you must have sweets, allow about 150 calories per day
for your favorite sweet – which amounts to roughly one ounce of chocolate, half a slice of cake, or 1/2 cup of ice cream.

Weight Control Tips & Secrets

99) It's a lot easier to eat 1,000 Calories than it is to burn 1,000 Calories by exercising. So a stroll after dinner won't offset the calories you ingest eating a big meal.

100) Understand that the only sure way to slim down for keeps is to eat less and exercise more. There are no safe short cuts or miracle methods for taking off weight.

101) Successful weight loss and subsequent weight maintenance requires knowledge, desire and discipline. Avoid the latest fad diets. Instead, take the time to develop a true understanding of weight control and then change your eating and activity habits accordingly.

Bonus Tips & Secrets

102) Consistently choose healthy foods, avoid harmful foods and large portions and exercise regularly. Nothing else will control your weight over the long haul.

103) Experts agree that whether you are trying to lose weight or just maintain your weight, it's calories that count. In theory it doesn't matter what foods the calories are from – to lose weight you must eat fewer calories than you burn.

104) Weight loss occurs when your food energy intake is less than the total energy you expend. This difference in calories is referred to as your calorie deficit.

105) How much weight you lose depends on the magnitude of your calorie deficit. To lose one pound requires a deficit of approximately 3,500 Calories.

106) Your body weight fluctuates two to three pounds daily. Your weight is lowest before breakfast and highest in the evening before retiring.

107) If you are overweight start on a weight loss diet now because it will only become more difficult to lose weight as you get older.

108) Inevitably, everyone on a diet hits a exasperating weight-loss plateau. The only way to bust through the plateau is to reduce your calorie intake and/or to step up your exercise intensity.

109) Slow weight loss is healthier, is more likely to be permanent, and is easier to sustain over the long haul. So when it comes to weight loss, don't be in a hurry!

110) The general weight-loss rule is "last on first off." When you lose weight, it normally it will come off in the reverse order of where you gained it. And there is not much you can do about that. There is no food, no exercise, no magic pill that will cause your body to lose fat in one place rather than another.

111) A very important weight-profile parameter is your waist-to-hip ratio. Health risks for heart attack and stroke increase considerably for men with a ratio above 1.0 and for women with a ratio above 0.8. To calculate your ratio, measure your waist size (at its narrowest circumference) and divide it by your hip size (at its widest section).

112) Handle occasional overeating by compensating. To do this, estimate how far you have strayed from your weight-loss diet and then make amends at the next opportunity (usually the next meal or two) – by eating less.

113) Eat the low-cal items on your plate first. Start with a broth soup, then the salad and veggies. By the time you get to the higher calorie meat and starch you'll be almost full and will eat less of them.

114) Studies show people who eat 5 to 6 mini-meals and snacks a day don't feel as hungry and are better able to control their appetite and their weight.

115) Fat-free isn't always your best bet. Low fat doesn't necessarily mean low calorie! Most often sugar is substituted for fat and the calorie total remains the same or even higher. Instead, look for low-calorie or reduced-calorie foods.

116) To prevent or delay the onset of type II diabetes, experts urge the overweight to lose weight and work out regularly. Weight loss helps your body use insulin more efficiently, and exercise helps metabolize excess circulating blood glucose.

117) Acquire a good low-calorie cookbook. Be sure the recipes cover breakfast, lunch and dinner, and all the recipes contain nutritional information, especially the number of calories per serving.

118) Obtain a comprehensive food calorie guide such as the excellent U.S.D.A. Home and Garden Bulletin No. 72:

"Nutritive Value of Foods," which can be downloaded at no cost.

119) Finally, get a scientifically sound and effective nutrition book to help you eat a safe and healthy manner. Consider NoPaperPress, with its extensive line of nutrition, weight control and exercise eBooks written by experts for sensible adults. No fads here! These are eBooks you can trust.

<u>**Related NoPaperPress™ eBooks**</u>

Eat Smart – U.S. Edition by Gail Johnson
Eat Smart – Metric Edition by Gail Johnson
Eat Smart – U.K. Edition by Gail Johnson

23

100-Day Super Diet-1200 Cal*	Weight Loss for Men - Metric*
100-Day Super Diet-1500 Cal*	Maximum Weight Loss- 1200 Cal*
100-Day No-Cooking Diet-1200 Cal*	Maximum Weight Loss- 1500 Cal*
100-Day No-Cooking Diet-1500 Cal*	Weight Control - U.S. Edition*
90-Day Smart Diet-1200 Cal*	Weight Control - Metric. Edition
90-Day Smart Diet-1500 Cal*	Prof Weight Control Women - U.S.
90-Day No-Cooking Diet - 1200 Cal*	Prof Weight Control Women - Metric
90-Day No-Cooking Diet - 1500 Cal*	Prof Weight Control Men - U.S.
90-Day Perfect Diet - 1200 Cal*	Prof Weight Control Men - Metric
90-Day Perfect Diet - 1500 Cal*	Weight Maintenance - U.S. Ed*
60-Day Perfect Diet-1200 Cal*	Weight Maintenance - Metric. Ed*
60-Day Perfect Diet-1500 Cal*	Weight Maintenance - UK Ed
50-Day Flex Diet-1200 Cal*	Weight Loss for Senior Men*
50-Day Flex Diet-1500 Cal*	Weight Loss for Senior Women*
30-Day Quick Diet - Women*	Eat Smart - U.S. Edition*
30-Day Quick Diet for Men*	Eat Smart - Metric Edition
30-Day No-Cooking Diet*	30-Day Mediterranean Diet
30-Day Diet - Women - Metric*	Exercise Smart - U.S. Edition*
30-Day Diet for Men - Metric*	Exercise Smart - Metric Edition
25 Day Easy Diet-1200 Cal*	Exercise Smart - UK Edition*
25 Day Easy Diet-1500 Cal*	Total Fitness - U.S. Edition
25-Day No-Cooking Diet	Total Fitness - Metric Edition
10-Day Express Diet	Total Fitness - UK Edition
10-Day No-Cooking Diet*	Total Fitness for Women-U.S. Ed*
7-Day Diet for Women*	Total Fitness for Women - Metric
7-Day Diet for Men*	Total Fitness for Women - UK Ed
7-Day No-Cooking Diets*	Total Fitness for Men - U.S. Ed*
90-Day Gluten-Free Diet-1200 Cal*	Total Fitness for Men- Metric Ed*
90-Day Gluten-Free Diet-1500 Cal*	Total Fitness for Men - UK Ed
30-Day Gluten-Free Quick Diet*	Senior Fitness - U.S. Edition*
30-Day Gluten-Free No-Cooking Diet*	Senior Fitness - Metric Edition*
7-Day Diet for Women - Metric*	Senior Fitness - UK Edition*
7-Day Diet for Men - Metric	Computer Diet - U.S. Edition*
7-Day Gluten-Free Express Diet*	Computer Diet - Metric Ed*
7-Day Gluten-Free No-Cooking Diet*	Reliable Weight Loss - U.S. Ed
90-Day Vegetarian Diet-1200 Cal*	101 Weight Loss Tips*
90-Day Vegetarian Diet-1500 Cal*	101 Healthy Eating Tips*
30-Day Vegetarian Diet*	101 Lifelong Fitness Tips*
7-Day Vegetarian Diet*	101 Weight Maintenance Tips
Weight Loss for Women*	101 Weight Loss Recipes
Weight Loss for Women - Metric	101 GF Weight Loss Recipes
Weight Loss for Women - UK	101 Veggie Weight Loss Recipes*
Weight Loss for Men*	30-Day Mediterranean Diet*
Maximum Weight Loss - 1200 Cal*	90-Day Mediterranean Diet - 1200 Cal*
Maximum Weight Loss - 1500 Cal*	90-Day Mediterranean Diet - 1500 Cal*

* These titles are available as both ebooks and paperbacks. Our ebooks are sold by Amazon, Apple, Google, Barnes & Noble and Kobo, but our paperbacks are only sold by Amazon.

<u>**Disclaimer**</u>

This work offers general Nutrition, weight control and exercise information. It is not a medical manual and the authors do not claim to be medically qualified. The material in this book is not intended to be a substitute for medical counseling. Everyone should have a medical checkup before beginning a weight control, or exercise program. Moreover, the physician conducting the medical exam should be made aware of and should approve the specific weight control or exercise program planned. Additionally, while the authors and publisher have made every effort to ensure the accuracy of the information in this book, they make no representations or warranties regarding its accuracy or completeness. Further, neither the authors nor publisher assume liability for any medical problems that might result from applying the methods in this book, or for any loss of profit, or any other commercial damages, including but not limited to special, incidental, consequential or other damages, and any such liability is hereby expressly disclaimed.